THE heart OF THE preacher

TO: DAN & SARAH,

I AM BLESSED TO BE YOUR PASTOR.
PRAYING DAILY FOR YOU.
GOD BLESS YOU!

YOUR PASTOR

III JOHN 2

Mirror press

THE heart OF THE preacher

James Crews

The Heart of the Preacher

Mirror Press
ISBN 0-89114-291-6

Printed in the United States of America

Dedication

To my wife, Jennifer, who has been my best friend for over 23 years. Without her this book would not have been completed.

Table of Contents

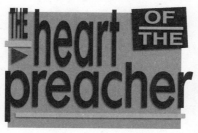

Foreword

Jesus spent much of His early ministry performing miracles in the lives of those who were ill from physical, mental or emotional diseases. It showed His concern for the well-being of those about Him. Much of the preacher's time today is involved in ministering to those who are ill. Whether it be visiting the hospital room, nursing home, or the home of the infirm, this is a way we can show our compassion for those who are ill.

In this effort to care for the flock, the shepherd often will allow himself to be attacked by the same diseases that attack the flock. We preachers will say, "It is better to wear out that to rust out." The fact of the matter is that God may not be pleased with either!

This book is an effort to encourage the preacher to be aware of ways he can care for himself. By doing this, he can be more effective for a much longer period of time. Heart disease is one thing which seems to have a big impact on preachers today.

As hospital chaplain, I have been caring for patients on the cardiac floors of our hospital for over ten years. But, recent chest pain and the resulting heart catheterization (including angioplasty) has given me a very different perspective on ministering to patients and their families.

I would encourage each person to read this book carefully and learn from the danger signals given, as well as the experience of the writer. I appreciate the effort that James Crews has put into compiling the information included in this book. I trust that it will help us to *"present our bodies a **living** (emphasis mine) sacrifice."*

Chaplain Phil Misenheimer
Washington Regional Medical Center
Fayetteville, Arkansas

Acknowledgements

For their assistance I want to thank:

The Portland Adventist Cardiac Rehabilitation Department for providing resource material and encouragement. I especially thank Sandi Dykes for her suggestions and words of encouragement.

The Southern Arkansas University Physical Education Department where I received my early training in health and fitness.

The Baptist Publishing House and Brother Larry Silvey for their willingness to print this material to aid our preachers.

My wife, Jennifer Crews, for proofing, editing, and typing my manuscript.

Our church member and friend, Cindy Miller, for completing our final manuscript on computer.

Brother Harold Hodges for his words of encouragement and letter detailing his personal experience of a cardiac event.

Heritage Baptist Church of Portland, Oregon, where I have the honor of serving as pastor. They have been tremendously understanding of me and have been used by the Lord to meet many of our needs especially since my heart attack and surgery.

Introduction

Heart attack! The very thought evokes a flood of emotional responses, especially to men in ministry — disability, unfulfilled God-given goals, grieving families, and denial. "It cannot or will not happen to me."

But the truth is, it can and does happen to approximately 1.5 million Americans yearly. Coronary heart disease is a silent killer and accounts for 500,000 deaths per year. That's more than cancer, AIDS, accidents, lung disease, and influenza combined.

Many men in the ministry are "walking time bombs" just waiting for a coronary artery to finally close off, thus permanently destroying portions, if not all, of their hearts.

As you read these words you have an amazing pumping machine at work in your chest. It is about the size of a closed fist and has been pumping at a steady rate of approximately 70 times per minute, 4,200 times per hour, and almost 37 million times per year. In a lifetime, it moves literally millions of gallons of blood (2,000 gallons per day) through its chambers, through the lungs, and to the furthest extremities of the human body. It is a miracle machine and the predominant organ in a *"fearfully and wonderfully made"* human body (Psalm 139:14). Why not pause right now and give God the glory for sustaining your life, saving your soul, putting you into the ministry (I Timothy 1:12).

Along with the privilege of physical life comes a corresponding responsibility to God, yourself, your family, and those whom God has called you to lead. Our spiritual life is our number one priority, but we must not shirk the responsibility of temple maintenance.

Having served full-time for over fifteen years as a church planter and pastor, I have never felt led, nor qualified, to write on theology or practical ministry. However, recently there has been a compelling urge in my heart to deal with the health issues of those who are serving God in the ministry. Initially, I considered entitling the book *Bodily Exercise Profiteth Little*, (I Timothy 4:8), emphasizing the first three words of that passage. But physical exercise is only one (though very important) facet of cardiovascular fitness.

Combined with my college degree (BSE in Physical Education and Biology), my experience as a former coach and science teacher, my years in ministry, and my recent heart attack and double by-pass surgery, I now feel somewhat qualified to speak on the subject of heart health.

More importantly, I want to be used by the Holy Spirit to motivate, encourage, and instruct those who have God's highest calling on their lives. Along with cardiovascular fitness comes the added dimension of an increased productivity, an overall sense of physical well-being, and the possibility of adding years to our lives. Of course, we all realize that our God is sovereign and controls the issues of life and death. But remember Jesus' rebuke to Satan when he said, *"Thou shalt not tempt the Lord thy God"* (Matthew 4:7). We would never gamble with our lives in foolish and sinful activity. Yet, countless numbers of preachers are gambling with their lives by unhealthy lifestyles. Remember the words of the apostle Paul in I Corinthians 6:19, 20. *"What? know ye not that **your body is the temple of the Holy Ghost** which is in you, which ye have of God, and **ye are not your own**? For ye are bought with a price: therefore **glorify God in your body**, and in your spirit, which are God's"* (Emphases mine).

If this book can influence one man of God to wake up and alter his lifestyle resulting in added years of a healthy, Spirit-led ministry, it will certainly be worth the time and effort invested in its completion.

Through the following pages we will be covering several crucial themes related to the heart of the preacher. I will do my best to condense as much material into one volume as possible. I know you don't have the time to sift through all the books and material as I am doing, so let me help. You will find illustrations and other important material to aid you in your quest for a healthy heart. So, if you are serious about your physical health and its implications to your ministry, read on and apply!

1

Serious as a Heart Attack

Monday, February 19, 1996, started as a typical day, but rapidly escalated into a turning point in my life. It was my day off and I had just completed a fairly vigorous exercise routine, including weight lifting and an aerobic video tape. By the conclusion of my aerobic workout I was feeling drained, somewhat sore, and out of breath. This should have been a warning, but I brushed it off as part of the aging process. For several months preceding this day, I had been feeling heavier and weaker while exercising and had been noticing a very slight pain in my chest.

But I had work to do! Without a rest from the workout, I immediately tackled a pile of bricks which needed relocating to the backyard. I felt this job could not wait another day or another minute. Taking the recycling container, I commenced to load it with bricks and made one trip after another. With each trip the pain in my chest intensified and my work slowed to a snail's pace. I was determined to go on until every brick was stacked in the designated place.

Having completed this *critical* task, I decided to take it easy the rest of the day. I assumed that the chest pain and overall discomfort would subside, but that thought quickly vanished. The feeling of weakness persisted and any activity brought another pain to the center of my chest.

Tuesday was an office day. Even though the symptoms hung on,

I drug myself out of bed and proceeded with my regular schedule of activity.

During this time my wife, Jennifer, was visiting Kari, our oldest daughter, while she was giving birth to our second grandchild. She was staying with her for a couple of weeks while I held down the fort with our other three children, Krista, Justin, and Jenna. I knew that if she had been home, she would have immediately taken me to the hospital. But my procrastination won out temporarily and I felt that what Jennifer didn't know wouldn't hurt her.

Wednesday morning brought no change, so I decided to visit the emergency room at a local hospital. To my astonishment it was painful to even walk across the parking lot and enter the emergency room door. After the preliminary paper work with the receptionist, I was ushered to a patient's cubicle and there waited for the doctor. After answering all the medical questions and having blood work, x-ray, and an electrocardiogram, the doctor gave his diagnosis. He said that I had pleurisy, which is an inflammation of the pleura, the membrane that covers the lungs. He prescribed rest and an anti-inflammatory drug. His prognosis was that in three to five days I should start to feel better and in seven to ten days I would be well. He placed no real restrictions or limitations on my physical activity.

The day passed, but the pain continued. (Did the doctor make a mistake?) I found it impossible to continue any exercise, walking, or weight lifting. Jennifer returned and she, too, was concerned. I met her insistence that I make a follow-up visit to my primary care doctor with firm resistance. I eventually yielded to her wishes.

The doctor did a general examination and studied my chest x-rays and the results of the previous tests. His only concern was a small spot on my lungs. He encouraged me to have a second x-ray after several months. He agreed with the emergency room doctor that because of my age, overall fitness, diet, and superficial test results, I was not the typical candidate for heart disease. But there was a flip side to the coin. My dad had died of a massive heart attack at age seventy. My personality could be characterized as *Type A*. And even with an altered diet, my cholesterol still hovered around 270.

My doctor's diagnosis was, "I'm not sure, but I don't think it's coronary heart disease." He prescribed a different type of anti-inflammatory pill and said, "Call back if you don't get better." Once again I received no restrictions or limitations on my activity.

Several more weeks passed and I experienced no improvement. I was planning to attend a church planting conference in Gary, Texas. Since I was serving as an interstate missionary, the national mission's department had provided me a round-trip airfare ticket and had made all the travel arrangements. I was very excited about the trip.

Jennifer felt very strongly that I should see a cardiologist before this trip. So a few days before my scheduled departure, I made an appointment with Dr. Mark Hart (how appropriate!), a cardiologist across the hall from my primary care doctor. Following his examination, he began making arrangements for a stress echocardiogram to be done. Though he did not seem overly concerned in the post examination conference, Jennifer and I began to wonder when he negotiated with some of the technicians to come in on their day off to perform this procedure. One nurse commented in passing that I must be a pretty special patient to receive this kind of urgent care. We began to question whether my condition was more serious than Dr. Hart had initially indicated.

The following Saturday morning I arrived bright and early for my stress echocardiogram. After being wired for the electrocardiogram, the technicians took computer enhanced images of my heart, including its chambers and coronary arteries. Then came the treadmill test. For several weeks my exertion level had been extremely low, but now I had to push it to the limit to get to the root of the problem. As the minutes passed and the treadmill speed increased, so did my pain. Peeking at the EKG readout to my left, I saw a very erratic-looking pattern. Dr. Hart put his arm on me and said "Just thirty more seconds." It felt like thirty minutes! Quickly I was rolled over onto the table and again an echocardiogram was taken.

Dr. Hart looked serious at the conclusion of the procedure and said it appeared very probable that I had coronary blockage and should have a cardiac catheterization immediately. After a couple of phone calls, the good doctor loaded me into a wheelchair and personally pushed me through a very long underground corridor to the main hospital.

This was the second cardiac catheterization of my life, so it held no surprises. During my college days a doctor in my hometown prematurely diagnosed me with possible heart disease. On that occasion my stay in Mercy Hospital in Miami, Florida, resulted only in a very large bill. This time, however, the report was bleak. During the catheterization, Dr. Hart pointed out on the monitor a completely blocked coronary artery and another major artery which allowed only a trickle of blood flow. Jennifer and I decided right then that I would go the route of open heart surgery. Hospital personnel then rolled me back to my room where I had to remain immobile for six hours.

All of that experience was pretty traumatic. The doctor informed me that I would miss my Texas trip and that I should refrain from preaching the next day. But the next day was our special *Friend Day*. Don't tell Dr. Hart, but I did preach to the largest crowd we have ever had. It also added an extra dimension to the service to inform the congregation that I was preaching against doctor's orders and would soon be facing double by-pass surgery. (This is not a recommendation to violate a doctor's orders.) I also had a colossal headache from the nitroglycerin patches placed on me during and following the previous day's treatment. God, however, blessed the service and gave me great liberty in preaching His Word. Souls were saved and our final count was 195 in attendance.

Between the time we received the test reports and the actual surgery, our lives certainly changed. I was not really fearful, but at times the thought of someone working on my heart through my open rib cage did give me the *creeps*. Those thoughts seemed to come especially strong just when I tried to get to sleep at night. Our entire family was now even more fat/cholesterol conscious. My exercise, which had been a regular part of my life for almost twenty-nine years, was now non-existent. Even showering brought on the angina pain which was an ever-present reminder of the up-coming surgery.

Dr. Hart put me in touch with Dr. John Lemmer, an excellent heart surgeon. He and his medical team perform over 1200 heart procedures each year. That was a great encouragement to me. During my initial interview with Dr. Lemmer, he showed Jennifer and me exactly what had to be done. The saphenous vein would be taken from the inside of my left leg and connected to the right side of my aorta. Then it would be attached to the posterior descending artery.

A mammary artery in the left side of my chest would also be rerouted to supply blood to the obtuse marginal artery which had 100 percent blockage. He reassured me that because of my age, health, and other factors I would be in the 99 percent survival group. "Even better than that!" he stated.

I wanted to wait until after Easter to have the operation, but Dr. Lemmer warned of the implications of such a delay. I was convinced and was placed on their schedule. The date was set — April 1, 1996.

The day finally arrived and I was looking forward to getting the surgery over with. We drove to Good Samaritan Hospital in downtown Portland and secured a place in their parking garage. While I was checking in, I received some strange looks from the people in the waiting area. My weight was 206 pounds and I appeared to be in good shape. They appeared to be surprised that I was being admitted for open heart surgery. Looks can be deceiving. All my tests the day before (blood pressure, lung capacity, iron level, pulse, etc.) said I was fine, but I was still a victim of coronary heart disease.

The volunteer who wheeled me to my room was a former corporate executive who had had a serious heart attack and by-pass surgery. He was in very good physical condition and gave me a pep talk about rehabilitation. Later he visited me following surgery.

The operating room was several hours behind schedule, which gave me time to get real *antsy*. Since I was a pastor, I had no pastor to visit me, but my good friend, Brother Mel Tittle, from Open Door Baptist Church filled those shoes. He took time on his day off to be a supportive friend. Brother Vernon Lee from Wyatt Baptist Church in El Dorado, Arkansas, also called me at least four times following the surgery. It's a blessing to have pastor friends you can lean on.

Soon I was prepared for surgery. (I didn't need all that hair anyway!) An intravenous line was inserted and I soon found myself in a room full of preoperative patients. A nurse removed my glasses which produced a blurry, dreamlike effect.

After about half an hour in the preoperative room, a nurse came to roll me the short distance to the operating room. The doors swung open and I saw probably ten masked doctors and nurses standing by an unbelievable amount of hi-tech equipment. The nurse parked the gurney parallel to the operating table and I was hoisted very quickly into place. One of the surgical nurses, commenting on my accent, asked me where I was from. We discovered that our home towns in Florida were only forty miles apart. That's the last thing I remember. Boy! Did the lights go out right in the middle of a sentence.

It would have been nice to have had a video tape of what took place in the next few hours. I cannot tell you what happened, but I will give you a brief layman's recital of this surgical procedure.

After the anesthesiologist places the patient into a deep sleep, the surgical team begins inserting a number of monitoring lines and devices into the patient's body. A breathing tube is placed through the trachea (windpipe) and into the lungs. A urinary catheter is inserted into the bladder for drainage and to monitor kidney function. Two additional lines are placed in the shoulder and wrist to monitor pressure in the arteries and veins and to withdraw needed blood samples.

One surgeon then begins to remove a portion of the saphenous vein from the leg. In my case the doctor made four one-inch incisions to remove it. The first cut was near the inside of the knee; the last was near the groin area. This vein's removal does not seem to hamper circulation in the leg as other veins take over its work.

While this leg work is being done, the chief heart surgeon begins his seven-inch vertical incision down the center of the chest. Once this has been done, the sternum is cut, separated, and held open by a metal retractor to allow the surgeons to perform their necessary procedures.

The heart is located in the pericardium which looks like a sack. The surgeon gently opens the pericardium and the beating heart is now exposed.

As quickly as possible the patient is placed on a heart-lung machine which takes over the work load of these vital organs. It's hard for me to comprehend the heart and lungs which have been steadily working since birth now taking a few hours of vacation.

Now it is time for the by-pass procedure. I had a double by-pass in which a small opening was made in my aorta (the main artery in the body which takes blood away from the heart). The vein taken from my leg was connected from this point to one of the coronary arteries which was nearly totally blocked. That's what is meant by the term *by-pass*. It by-passes the blockage to bring blood to the deprived area.

My second by-pass rerouted the left internal mammary artery which comes from the aorta and supplies blood to the chest wall. Now it is routed to the obtuse marginal artery, an area which had 100 percent blockage and where a mild heart attack had taken place. Once the by-pass is proven secure, the patient is taken off the pump and, hopefully, the heart will begin beating on its own. Sometimes, however, a slight shock must be administered to the heart before it regains its normal function.

Before the chest is closed, two large plastic tubes are inserted about two inches below the main incision in order to drain any post-operative blood from the heart and chest area. These tubes are removed a couple of days after surgery.

Then the breastbone is brought back together and secured with several strands of stainless steel wire. These will be a permanent part of the patient's anatomy. The skin is then sutured and covered with a sterile dressing.

With the operation completed, the patient will soon awake in the recovery room. I recall this experience fairly well. Because of the strong medication, I felt very little pain. When I was sufficiently awake, I was informed that all went well. Later, Jennifer made her first visit. As she entered the room, the nurses were completing a clean up job required because I had rather violently removed an intravenous needle. She said I was pretty "goofy" and even blew a kiss at her when she left. I also motioned for her to feel free to go on home and get some rest.

My thoughts of *this isn't so bad* began to fade as the pain set in. Open heart surgery is not a piece of cake in spite of what you may have heard. I have had several broken bones, bruised kidneys, two knee operations, and other injuries, but nothing compares to the way I felt following this surgery. Maybe I just have a low pain tolerance or maybe I'm just not tough, but, friend, you do not want to go through this procedure.

As I write this account, I have forgotten some of the pain experiences much like the example of a woman in travail forgetting her pain (John 16:21), but I certainly will never forget all the pain and discomfort of the ensuing days.

Very soon after surgery, the critical care nurse had me sit on the side of my bed, dangle my feet, and even cough! That was no fun. I became nauseated as soon as I sat up. I began to gag which brought on tremendous pain in my chest. She helped me back into bed to my great relief. Breathing exercises and coughing were to be a part of my daily schedule. I dreaded every minute of it. Removing my chest tubes brought serve pain as did the removal of the three wires in the lower portion of my incision.

I haven't missed my personal devotional time in years, but Jennifer had to read for me the day following surgery. For several days following surgery, I had to force myself just to read a daily portion of the Word of God and rush through my prayer list. Jennifer had bought me the book *Experiencing God* before my hospital stay, but it lay on the table beside me unopened until my trip home.

I could go on about the horrors of open heart surgery, but I hope you get the picture. Without question, God had a divine purpose in this situation and I believe my spiritual growth was real during this time. So in many cases I would not change what happened. I intentionally brought out the negative side to motivate you to take care of yourself so you will increase your chances of avoiding this ordeal.

The following chapters will examine, step by step, some practical habits you can develop to reduce the possibility of having a cardiac event. They will also encourage you to develop some lifestyle changes which I believe will bring glory to God.

Preachers at Risk

Observe those around you the next time you are around a group of preachers. We come in all shapes and sizes and by the very nature of our calling, we are *preachers at risk*. Most God-called pastors and other full-time Christian workers live very sedentary, yet highly stressful lives. Our diets usually leave much to be desired, and exercise ranks very low on our list of priorities. Of course, I am speaking in general terms, but I'm sure you agree with the preceding generalities.

Pastors may also be characterized by several other common denominators. First, you are disciplined. By definition, a disciple is a disciplined one, an ardent non-compromising follower of Jesus Christ. This God-inspired discipline can and should be channeled into other areas of your life. Your health should be one of these areas.

Second, you are highly motivated. Because of God's calling on your life you have an external and, more importantly, an internal motivating power peculiar to a child of God. With that in mind, consider your responsibility to your physical well-being.

Third, you are obedient. If anyone is obedient, it should be God's prophets. Without question, I believe the Holy Spirit will lead you to take better care of His temple if you will only listen. Our only recourse is to obey that prompting. Yes, we may be at risk, but we have the tools to tip the scales in our favor in the area of a healthy heart.

Risk factors may be defined as conditions and habits (many of which are of our own making) which increase the likelihood of developing coronary heart disease. A good, working understanding of those risk factors can be extremely helpful in heading off potential heart problems.

According to nearly every resource, risk factors fall into two major categories: those factors you cannot change and those factors you can change. While some things are beyond our capacity to alter, there are also those risk factors which could, with relatively basic lifestyle changes, impact our health dramatically.

This chapter will put a spotlight on those two categories especially in regard to the preacher. First, let's consider risk factors you cannot change. As much as you may try, you can do nothing to erase these three factors — your age, your sex, and your heredity.

Age. Of course, there are only two alternatives to aging: death and the Rapture! Let's face it, the more years that pass, the more likely we are to face some type of cardiac event. It's always an encouragement to see older preachers still fearlessly preaching the Word, but along with those additional years comes a greater chance of clogged arteries. The condition usually begins early in life, but becomes progressively worse with advanced age. Aging is an unchangeable risk factor.

Sex. Risk factor number two is your sex. Statistically, men have a higher rate of coronary heart disease when compared to those weaker vessels we call women. Rates of heart disease in women do, however, begin to catch up with men with the onset of menopause and are almost equal with men by the age of sixty.

Heredity. Unchangeable risk factor number three is heredity. We didn't choose our parents and from them and other relatives there comes a certain combination of genes. If you have immediate family members who had heart problems at relatively young ages, you are at a greater risk of developing problems yourself.

Another factor under family risk is childhood family environment. Contributing factors in this area would be parents who smoke, a high fat/cholesterol childhood diet, and high levels of stress in the home. Those are things in the past and, of course, cannot be changed. However, there may be damage done during our formative years which is completely beyond our ability to change.

The second major category of risk factors covers those areas which may be modified or eliminated completely through needed lifestyle changes. These include smoking, high cholesterol, high blood pressure, being overweight, lack of exercise, improper stress management, and diabetes.

I often tell people "There are two things which promote the sin of worry. First, those things which we cannot change and second, those things we can change. If we cannot change them, why worry? If we can change them, let's set out to do so." The same prescription goes for cardiac risk factors. Let's set out to change what we can by the grace and power of God.

I had a heart attack and by-pass surgery. I may have a repeat of those events. But, I do not want to stand before God and have to admit that I did not do everything possible to eliminate every potential risk factor. What about you? With this in mind, let's examine these potentially hazardous factors in our lives which we can do something about. Later we will examine in more detail the Big Three: exercise, diet, and stress.

Smoking. I debated about how to present this obvious risk factor. So here I go. God's spokesmen should not smoke! It's a sin against the body and a nasty habit which should not once be named among the child of God, let alone the man who stands in the pulpit. Even most lost people know smoking is wrong. But I know that some preachers do smoke and even justify it. Whether you agree with my philosophy or not, there's one thing that's certain. Smoking (all forms of tobacco) affects your heart and blood vessels. There is substantial evidence that smoking is one of the most destructive forms of self-gratification on this planet. People who smoke a pack of cigarettes a day have twice the risk of heart attack as non-smokers.

If you smoke, by the help of the Lord Jesus, purpose to stop. If you don't smoke, don't ever start. It may not be easy, but an application of Philippians 4:13 is certainly appropriate here. This decision, like any other commitment to the Lord, will not be regretted. You'll be glad you did!

Cholesterol. Cholesterol is a fatty, yellow, wax-like substance found in animal tissue and normally present in the blood. It is also naturally manufactured by the liver. Cholesterol is found in many of America's favorite foods — eggs, dairy products, and meat. Your body does need this substance to some degree, but most people (especially preachers) ingest far too much. In the chapter on diet you will find more detail about consuming too much fat and cholesterol. In addition to consuming too many high fat foods, your cholesterol can be increased by lack of exercise and high stress which produces an excessive flow of adrenalin. Too much cholesterol allows a buildup of harmful deposits in the arterial walls and results in atherosclerosis (hardening of the arteries). This condition can lead to heart attacks and strokes.

It is important to know your cholesterol numbers. A total cholesterol of 200 is about borderline for most people. For people with other risk factors the cholesterol count should be lower. In addition to your total cholesterol count you should learn your LDL (low density lipoprotein), also know as "bad" cholesterol, and your HDL (high density lipoprotein) or "good" cholesterol. Your doctor or cardiologist, as well as others, can administer these periodic tests and evaluate your results. Please don't put off this important step.

Some people cannot lower their cholesterol by traditional means and must resort to prescribed medication. I am presently on one of these drugs and my total cholesterol was lowered by 97 points in a four-month period. Prior to this, nothing seemed to affect my cholesterol count. These drugs may cause side effects, but, thank the Lord, my medication has caused none.

Blood Pressure. What is your blood pressure? When was the last time you had it checked? With the wide-spread availability of blood pressure measuring devices at our disposal, we have no excuse for not knowing. Many of these machines are free of charge and are, for the most part, fairly accurate. Classification of blood pressure readings are usually prominently displayed for comparison.

Hypertension or high blood pressure is simply an excessive amount of pressure on the arteries. It increases the chance of atherosclerosis by allowing plaque to build up in the arterial walls. High blood pressure is linked to congestive heart failure, strokes, and kidney failure. It also increases the work load of the heart. It is a silent killer with few recognizable symptoms.

Again, the remedy is primarily found in lifestyle changes. Weight loss, regular exercise, reduced stress, and a reduction of salt can all contribute to lowering the blood pressure. Medication may also be required for some individuals.

Weight. Approximately 30 percent of the American population has the distinction of being 20 percent above a designated, desirable body weight. I wonder where we preachers fit in with those stats. Excess baggage on the body intensifies other risk factors such as high blood pressure, elevated blood cholesterol, and diabetes. Too much fat tissue makes the heart work harder, thus hindering the supply of blood and oxygen to the rest of the body. Following my surgery I lost twenty pounds and it surely makes a difference.

The key to weight loss is to gradually lose weight by eating less calories and fat and burning more through a regular exercise program. The next two chapters will have more detail about these desirable lifetime commitments.

It's not easy to lose those excess pounds that took a lifetime to accumulate, but it can and should be done. With so many delicious fat-free and reduced-calorie foods available, there's really no excuse not to make some changes. Our entire family has made great strides in a healthy diet plan, and the results have shown up on the scales!

Exercise. The American Heart Association ranks physical inactivity as number four in contributing risk factors for coronary heart disease. According to the Public Health Service, "Forty percent of adult Americans are sedentary." Only 20 percent of our population exercises vigorously on a regular basis. Another source stated that inactive people are 1.9 times more likely to suffer from heart disease. Is lack of exercise a risk? You better believe it is! When you omit regular exercise from your schedule, you are in turn missing out on a host of benefits. Those benefits include a stronger, more efficient heart, greater muscle tone, and increased endurance and energy. The next chapter will focus on exercise.

Stress. Stress is a part of normal living and a certain amount of it is needful. It could be defined as "mental or physical tension; urgency, pressure, etc." The body's reaction to stress, when properly managed can be a real plus, but mismanaged stress can be deadly. Inability to cope with a stressful situation can become *distress* and in turn cause some pretty serious physiological problems. The adrenal glands begin to work resulting in a rise in blood pressure as well as heart rate. The blood vessels begin to constrict and cholesterol levels begin to go up.

Most preachers probably would be described as Type A personalities. Some characteristics of a Type A are desirable; others are not. If we are marked by impatience, unbiblical anger, and even hostility, we have a spiritual problem as well as a dangerous physical condition. We should identify our stressful areas and seek to alter our attitudes toward godly solutions. Chapter five will discuss the problems of stress.

Diabetes. It has been estimated that approximately fourteen million Americans have diabetes. If you are one of those, you are at greater risk for developing coronary heart disease. Elevated blood sugar can be brought under control by diet and exercise, however, some individuals must take oral medication or injections of insulin to regulate the glucose level in the body. If you have a family history of diabetes or if you have heart disease, you should monitor your sugar level.

Well, there you have it — a total of ten risk factors. Some are beyond our control. Others are controllable and in many cases can be eliminated. Next we will consider the three most important steps to promote a healthy heart. Regular exercise, proper diet, and stress management could give you the one-two-three punch for a strong healthy body. So, with a willing heart ask the Holy Spirit to speak to you about what He would have you to do.

CHAPTER 3

Bodily Exercise Profiteth

Some may accuse me of pulling I Timothy 4:8 out of context for this chapter's title. Let me assure you, that is not my intention. But I am thoroughly convinced that bodily exercise or physical training is, in God's sight, beneficial and, in fact, necessary for this earthly tabernacle. There is a direct correlation between emotional and spiritual health and the health of the body. If this be true, physical fitness should occupy a portion of our daily schedules. Of course, I am not implying that bodily exercise can even come close to a state of godliness; that the verse makes abundantly clear. But let's not "throw out the baby with the bath water." Face it, Preacher, in the "here and now" physical conditioning is important. Amen? Now that we've got that settled, let's move on.

In most cultures of the past and up until recent decades, no one had to harp on physical fitness. It was included in their very lifestyle. People of past generations, as a whole, walked more, ate a more nutritious diet, and had a handle on stress management even though they didn't know today's lingo or the benefits of their actions.

The Industrial Revolution brought a drastic decline in physical activity. Mechanical power has replaced man power, and the result has been one of the most sedentary civilizations in the history of the world.

Full-time Christian workers, especially pastors, have a distinct advantage over nearly every other profession. We can usually set our schedules according to our priorities. Our personal walk with God should occupy first place. Our families must never be neglected and we must perform our ministries with excellence. All these areas must fit the schedule of our waking hours. We always have the time for what's important. Isn't that what we all preach? But what about "temple" maintenance? Surely we can find a few minutes per day to devote to physical conditioning.

My own lifetime commitment to exercise began in November of 1967. From that time until the present, exercise has been an important part of my life. Through high school, college, coaching and teaching days, as well as my twenty years in full-time ministry, physical training has been a continuing project. The only interruptions were for surgeries or for other unexpected major occurrences. I definitely strive to "practice what I preach" in this chapter.

In this chapter we will examine several topics including the benefits of exercise, types of exercise, and some basic guidelines on how to begin a consistent exercise program.

Benefits

According to Dr. Brown, my college anatomy and physiology teacher, there are approximately 792 muscles and 206 bones in the human body. *The Complete Life Encyclopedia* by Minirth and Meier says we have ten billion nerve cells and over 60,000 miles of blood vessels. With a complex machine such as ours, we better keep it in tip-top shape.

Few authorities would debate the obvious benefits of a fit body. Much research has gone into the benefits of exercise, though the jury is still out concerning some of the claims resulting from those studies. However, if a majority of these benefits results from regular exercise, it would do us all well to be willing to begin, continue, or intensify our exercise programs.

Cardiovascular fitness is universally believed to be an observable and predictable benefit of regular exercise training. Your heart is a high-tech muscle which must be exercised to remain strong. Regular exercise not only builds the heart, but other muscles as well. Our skeletal muscles, properly worked, will strengthen our bodies giving us more stamina and an overall sense of well-being. And remember this — muscles use more calories than do fat cells. We can control our weight, improve our digestion, and sometimes even suppress our appetites as a result of exercise training. Exercise also can improve our sleep, decrease stress, and lower high blood pressure. It can lower our chances of a heart attack or a second one. Exercise can be a very enjoyable diversion from a hectic schedule and, to some, it can become a very profitable hobby. Yes, there are many benefits to regular exercise.

Three Types of Exercise

I will cover three types of exercise in the following pages. In order to operate at peek efficiency, you should include all three in your training schedule. They are stretching, aerobics, and weight training.

Stretching. Stretching is easy to learn and can be done in a minimum amount of time. Stretching benefits all ages, but is especially important as we age due to the increased loss of elasticity in our tendons and muscles. Flexibility serves as a deterrent to muscle and joint injuries, and it just plain feels good! Your stretching can be a significant part of your warming up and cooling down activities. Your exercises should be performed slowly and easily without bouncing and without pain.

Preceding your aerobics or weight training, stretching will increase the blood flow to the targeted muscles and prepare them for their work. Allow at least three to five minutes for this phase of your exercise program. If you choose to stretch for longer periods of time, that is even better. Just remember to take enough time to enjoy all the aforementioned benefits and prevent the possibility of overtaxing your cardiovascular system.

Your cool down period is just as important as your warm up. If you stop exercising abruptly, there is the danger of blood "pooling" in the extremities, especially the legs. This can result in a reduced flow of return blood to the heart causing dizziness and even fainting. So take the time (three to five minutes) to cool down. Cool down activities can include the stretching exercises along with slow walking.

I have included several suggested stretching techniques in this chapter. You may choose several or all of these according to your time and exercise program. It is especially important to stretch the large muscle groups in your legs, because they utilize the most blood and will probably carry the brunt of your aerobic exercise.

As you perform each stretch, start slowly with only mild tension. Hold for several seconds, and once the tightness subsides, move slightly more into the stretch until you feel a mild pull. Remember to refrain from bouncing and do not overextend the stretching motion. It should be a relaxed exercise focusing on the muscles being stretched. Maintain normal and controlled breathing. When you have concluded your stretching exercises, move immediately into the next phase of your workout.

Aerobics. Aerobic exercise is by far the most important part of your fitness program. *Aerobics* means "with oxygen" and is any type of exercise which steadily supplies sufficient amounts of oxygen to the affected muscles throughout the exercise period. It is a sustained exercise that keeps the heart rate elevated. Aerobics training utilizes large muscle groups in continuous motion. To obtain optimal results, your aerobics exercise program should be the proper frequency, duration, and intensity. We will examine each of these three factors later.

Some exercises would not qualify as aerobic, though they may be helpful in other ways. These *anaerobic* exercises would include golf, weight lifting, softball, volleyball, etc. These exercises certainly are good, but they do not maintain a high level of activity to improve endurance and true cardiovascular fitness.

So, Preacher, find an exercise to get you moving and keep you moving. Better yet, pick more than one type of aerobic exercise for variety. Find something you enjoy or you won't keep it up for the long haul. Be consistent, and that doesn't mean every other Saturday or only during nice weather!

There are many forms of aerobic exercises from which to choose. Before you begin this lifestyle change though, you should visit your doctor for a full physical exam and his recommendation, especially if you have been living a sedentary life or if you have one or more risk factors mentioned in chapter two. Also remember to start at a low level of intensity and gradually build.

I will suggest some forms of aerobic exercises and talk about my favorite one, walking, last.

Suggestion #1   Jogging or Running

Running gives the fastest and most intense aerobic workout. It is very popular, requires no special equipment other than proper footwear, and, of course, burns a lot of calories. However, running causes a lot of stress and strain on lower body bones and joints and is an easy *burn-out* activity.

Suggestion #2   Cycling

Many people choose cycling because it is very enjoyable and is not as stressful on the joints as jogging and running. Cycling can be done outdoors and, during inclement weather, indoors (stationary bike) and is an excellent lower body conditioner.

Suggestion #3 Swimming

Swimming works all the major muscle groups and many believe it to be the best total conditioning workout possible. But few people have year-around access to a swimming facility, and swimming must be continuous to be classified as a true aerobic exercise.

Suggestion #4 Aerobic classes

Many people who enjoy the motivation of working out in groups find exercise classes very popular. Aerobic tapes are also available for use at home. But, as with all other forms of exercise, remember the importance of warming up, cooling down, and staying within your heart's target rate.

Suggestion #5 Walking

Walking is by far the safest, easiest, and most convenient form of aerobic exercise. You can walk almost anywhere and it does not require costly equipment, other than a good pair of walking shoes. When done correctly, walking will increase cardiovascular fitness and take off weight. Brisk walking burns approximately 350 calories an hour. The American Heart Association estimates that a 200-pound person, with no change in diet, could lose fourteen pounds in one year by walking briskly each day for one and one-half miles. This most natural form of exercise is probably the easiest to monitor with respect to time, distance, and pulse rate. Non-athletes, overweight people, and people suffering from heart disease all can benefit greatly from this simple activity.

My wife and I enjoy walking five to six days per week. It gives us a great opportunity to be together and to talk. We live in Portland, Oregon, which has more days of measurable precipitation than almost any other major city in America, yet we still keep walking in our schedules. Our typical walk takes place on Powel Butte, located three blocks from our home. It is a 570 acre volcanic mound with over nine miles of rugged, rarely flat trails. It is a beautiful place and has been described by one journalist as a microcosm of the state of Oregon. I realize you may not have such a perfect setting readily accessible for your exercise walking, but walking can be done almost anywhere!

One of my pastor friends, also a heart by-pass survivor, walks two miles per day, five to six days per week in the flat lands of Oklahoma. He and his wife always hold hands and talk.

In exercise walking, as in other forms of aerobic conditioning, footwear is very important. Take the time to find the *right* shoe for you. There are several shoes on the market designed just for walking. They are lightweight, pliable, and offer good arch support. The padded heal takes the impact of continuous walking. If you walk in a wooded area, a good pair of low-cut hiking boots would be a good investment.

When you walk, stand straight and start slow. Stride heel to toe and allow your arms to swing naturally. Breathe deeply and after you have walked a few minutes, pick up the pace. You may also want to include some short bursts of activity during your walk. Examples may be quicker strides, hills, stairs, or jumping jacks. Studies reveal that these short bursts of high intensity activity help burn more calories and aid in total conditioning. *But don't overdo it!*

Other forms of aerobic exercises could include handball, tennis, racquetball, skating, or even mowing the yard. Just remember to get moving and keep moving.

The frequency of an aerobic program varies with the individual. To reap any significant benefits, however, it should be performed at least three times per week. If this is your goal, you will probably want to exercise on alternate days. Once you become accustomed to your routine, you may want to increase to four, five, or even six times per week. The Lord's fourth commandment certainly applies here. I never walk seven days a week. Five to six days should be the maximum; three should be the minimum. Just three days per week will make a substantial difference in your heart and fitness level.

Twenty- to sixty-minute sessions are recommended to maintain cardiovascular fitness and to burn calories. This does not count your warm-up and cool-down activities. For beginners who are out of shape, the duration of exercise can vary. Just listen to your body. You may have to start with five- to ten-minute sessions and gradually increase over time. A gradual progression in your training will also help you avoid injury and decrease the chance for sore muscles and joints.

The intensity of your exercise period is very important. How hard you train will be determined by your heart's target range. Exercising below your target rate will gain few benefits. Exercising above this range increases the possibility of heart complications and bone injuries. You may need to consult a physician or, better yet, a competent cardiologist to help in determining your own target range. This can be done through a treadmill stress test. Following this test your doctor can prescribe a personal target rate for you.

If you do not choose to consult a physician regarding your exercise intensity, there is a simple formula you can use to determine your heart rate. This is just a formula which applies to most people, so please use caution. First, subtract your age from 220. This will represent your maximum heart rate. Then take 75 percent of that number to get your ideal exercise heart rate. For example, I am 44. Subtracting that number from 220 leaves 176. That's my maximum heart rate. Then, multiplying that total by .75 gives me 132. So 132 would be a target rate to maintain during the aerobic portion of my workout. Here's the formula again: 220 - your age X .75 = your target rate. Seventy-five percent is an ideal target rate. Anything under 60 percent will yield minimal benefits. Anything over 85 percent could be potentially dangerous, unless you are in condition to exercise at peak athletic performance. So try to keep your aerobics between 60 and 85 percent of your maximum. For me that would be between 105 and 149.

To check your heart rate, take your pulse by placing two fingers over your carotid artery (located on the side of your throat), or at the wrist just below the base of the thumb. Count the number of beats for fifteen seconds and then multiply by four.

It's good to take your pulse before, during, and at the cool-down stage of your exercise. After some time of consistent training you will be able to judge your level of exercise. But it's always wise to periodically check your heart rate just to know for sure. For my last birthday, Jennifer gave me a heart rate monitor. This device is perfect to help me stay in my heart rate zone.

Thus far, we have covered stretching to stay loose and flexible, and aerobics to get the blood flowing and oxygen levels up. Now let me say a word about weight lifting.

Weight Lifting

Weight lifting, or resistance training as it is now defined, will offer considerable benefits to your body if done correctly. Johns Hopkins School of Medicine, as well as other prestigious medical schools, has conducted a great deal of research on the benefits of moderate weight training. As a result, many experts now recommend that you add weight lifting to your aerobic workout. I am not advocating weight training as a substitute, but rather as a supplement to your total exercise program.

While there is still some debate on this subject, there is also general agreement that weight training may contribute the following benefits:

• It strengthens the heart muscle while reducing fat cells throughout the body.

• It increases cardiovascular endurance by building muscle mass in the arms and legs.

• It lowers blood pressure as well as antihypertensive medications do.

• It keeps bones stronger and more dense; this protects against injury.

• It increases levels of HDL (good cholesterol) as well as aerobics do.

• It aids in controlling diabetes and for some may even eliminate the symptoms of Type II non-insulin diabetes.

• It increases physical strength, thus making the normal demands of life easier to handle.

• It can be continued regardless of age. It will increase strength and flexibility substantially in older adults if done consistently.

So, Preacher, start pumping the iron. You'll be glad you did. I began a serious weight training program in 1967 (before it was fashionable) and have, through the years, attempted to learn as much as possible on the subject. I have also designed weight lifting programs for individuals and supervised the weight programs for our junior and senior high football teams while I was coaching. New research has caused me to discard some of my earlier philosophies, but my basic theories have remained the same.

Let me now attempt to answer some questions about effective resistance training.

How often should you lift weights? For a basic fitness program, two or three days per week is ideal. Two days will give the muscle tone maintenance needed, and three days will result in significant gains. Weight training should also be done on alternate days, such as Monday, Wednesday, and Friday or Tuesday, Thursday, and Saturday. Before my heart surgery, I worked out two days a week and walked three. Now I work out three days on the weights and walk five to six days. I have made tremendous progress in strength and endurance because of these increases.

How should I lift? First, your program should begin with adequate stretching and warming up. You will reduce your risk of injury by starting slowly and easily. Breathing is another concern. An old technique I used was to hold my breath until I was about ready to pop, then exhale at the peak of the lift. That's not advisable. Breathing should be deep, but not held. Begin the lift with a full breath of air and *blow* the weight up, exhaling throughout the lift. Follow the return stage by gathering in another breath of air. It should feel natural and comfortable. Remember, a beet-red face and nearly passing out does not equate with proper breathing.

Your basic lifts should be performed through a *full range of motion,* concentrating on the muscle groups being worked. Also check your posture so as not to cause back injury or muscle strain.

How much should you lift? The amount of weight to use in your lifting varies greatly with the type of exercise you are doing as well as your own physical condition. After experimenting with each exercise (preferably under supervision), you can establish your maximum amount for each lift. Please be careful. Start with light weights and gradually work up to heavier lifts. Once you determine your maximum, you can then use 30 to 40 percent of this total for your target weight. With this amount you can probably accomplish ten to fifteen repetitions. One series of these lifts is called a *set.* A good goal is three sets of ten to fifteen repetitions of each exercise. To increase muscle mass and strength, lower your repetitions and increase your weight load.

Make sure you rest between sets for about a minute. As your physical condition improves, you can reduce your rest time to fifteen to twenty seconds between sets.

What kind of weights should you use? Through the years I have lifted *free weights* (barbells and dumbbells) and I have used various types of machines. Each type has certain advantages and benefits. Free weights are less expensive and they work certain muscle groups in a way not equaled by machines. Machines, on the other hand, are simpler, quieter, and less messy than a bunch of loose weights and bars. A couple of months following my by-pass, I purchased a Wieder Weight Machine. It was on sale for less than $300.00. (Good treadmills are much higher than that.) I have been very pleased with this sharp looking piece of equipment. It has stations which efficiently work every muscle group and can be used by our entire family. When I first bought the machine, my bench press weight was at a minimum. Six months following surgery I bench pressed 210 pounds. That gives you an idea of how fast strength can be gained through a good program.

To conclude these three phases of exercise, I will share with you my workout schedule. I do not intend to extend the length of these workouts, so you can consider them my ultimate training program.

- Warm up and stretching (daily) - 5 to 7 minutes.
- Weight training (3 days per week) - 15 to 20 minutes.
- Exercise walking (5-6 days per week) - 30 to 45 minutes.
- Cool down and stretching (daily) - 3 to 5 minutes.

It is my prayer that this section on exercise has helped you develop your own program. Remember, we are all different and have varied schedules, but please include exercise in that schedule!

Here are some precautions and guidelines on safe exercise which I have found helpful.

• Seek a doctor's advice before starting your exercise program. Better to be safe than sorry!

• Set realistic goals. Don't push yourself by doing too much too soon. Listen to your body and don't overdo it. If you become fatigued, it's okay to rest.

• Be consistent with your exercise program, but if you miss a day don't worry. Get back on schedule and strive to continue exercising for a lifetime. Reward yourself when you reach your goals.

• Choose the best time for you. Pick the time of day when your energy level is high.

• Pick one or more aerobic exercises for variety. Make sure you can exercise year-round.

• Work out with your wife, children, or others. A training partner guarantees accountability and motivation.

• Wear proper clothing for current weather conditions. Don't overdress on hot, humid days. Natural fibers like cotton rather than spandex or rubber allow for evaporation of sweat. Wear several layers in cold weather and remove layers as needed. Protect your head and face. Most of your heat loss comes from these areas. Wear proper footwear.

• Do aerobics and weight training on proper surfaces. Always use equipment as directed.

• Do not hold your breath or strain excessively. Rhythmic, deep breathing is the key.

• Drink plenty of water before and after working out.

• Wait one to two hours after a heavy meal before exercising.

• Stop exercising if you experience any of the following: chest, arm, or jaw discomfort; shortness of breath; change of heart rate (rapid, irregular, or flutters); dizziness; faintness; nausea; or excessive fatigue.

• Always remember your warm up, cool down, and stretching.

• Take added precautions against injury.

Preacher, I've done my part; the ball's in your court! Remember, "Bodily exercise profiteth." You'll not regret a commitment to health and physical fitness.

Bench press

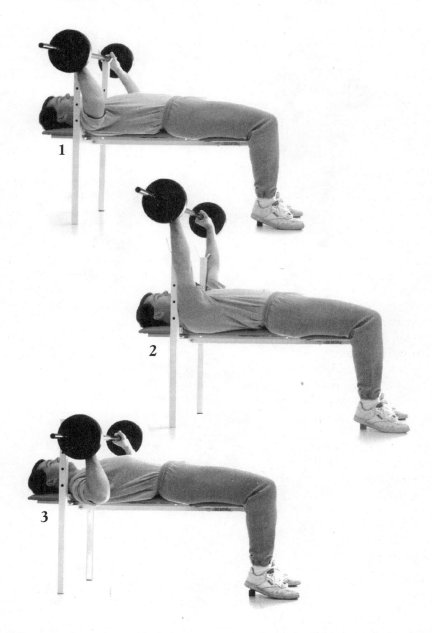

Military press

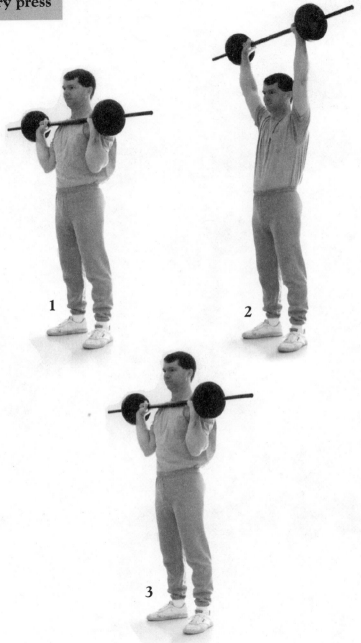

Squats

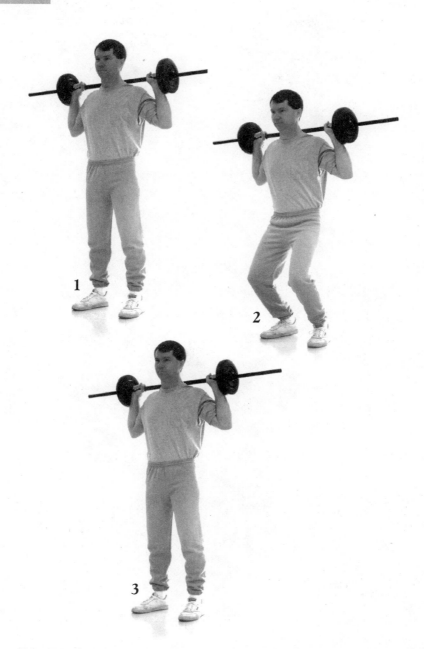

Toe raises

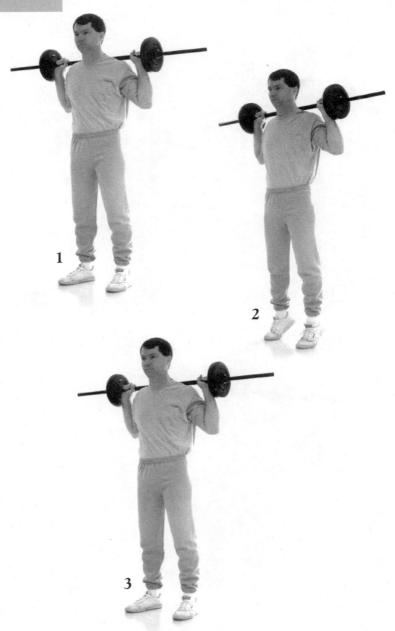

Tricep press

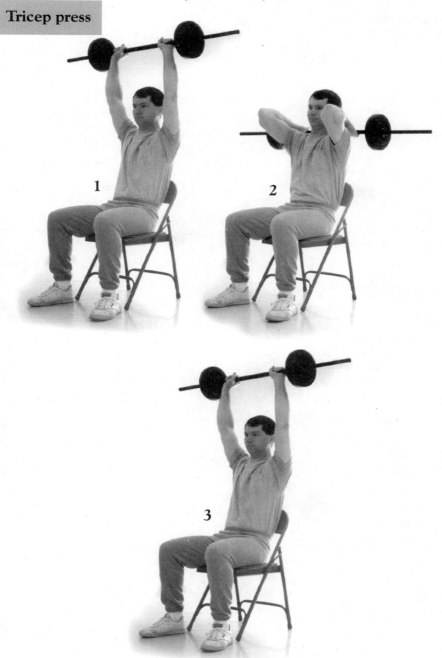

Upright rowing

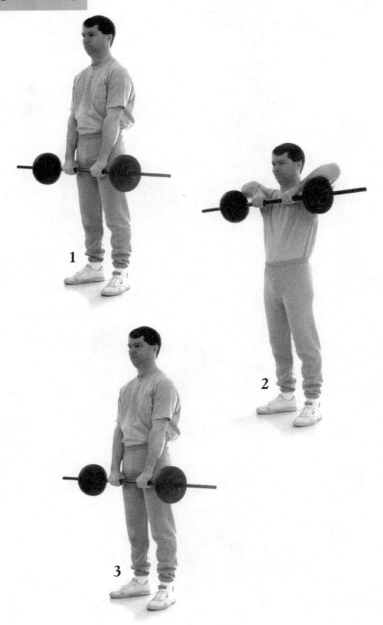

Standard bicep curl

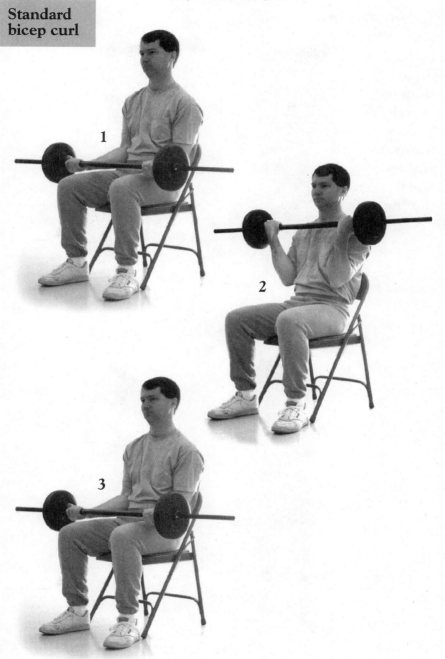

Tricep stretch

Include these stretching exercises in your warm-up and cool-down routine.

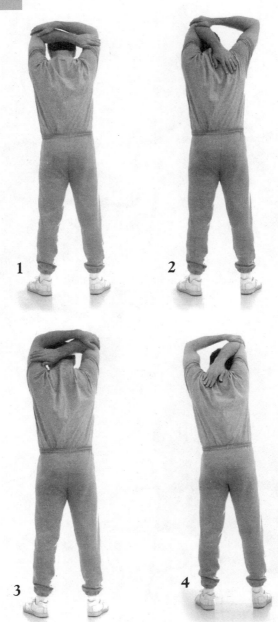

1

2

3

4

Tricep stretch provides flexibility to triceps and the top of shoulders.

Side arm stretch

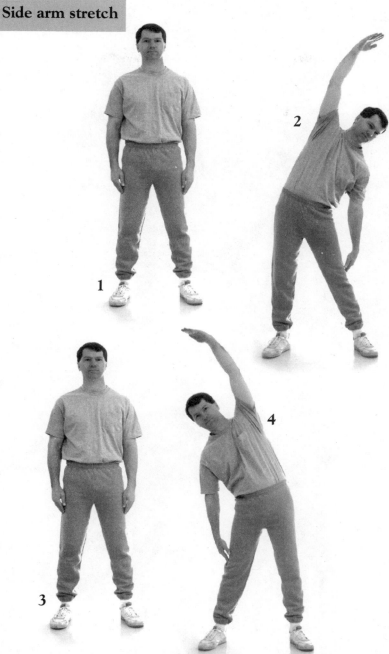

Side arm stretch provides flexibility to the muscles on the side.

Front thigh stretch

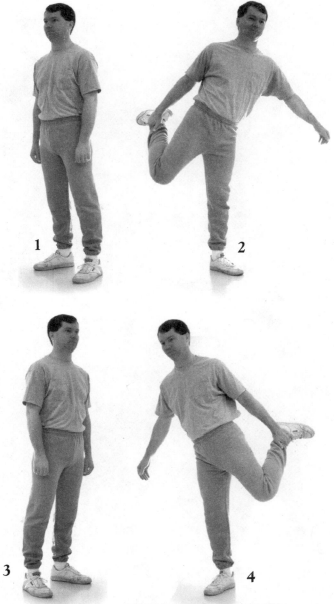

Front thigh stretch prepares muscles on the front upper leg.

Fencer stretch

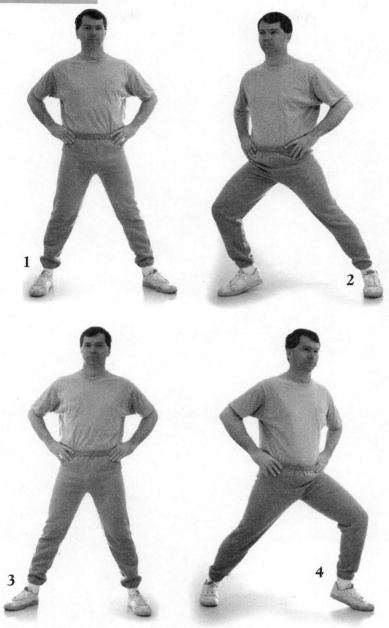

Fencer stretch prepares muscles of the inner leg.

Calf stretch

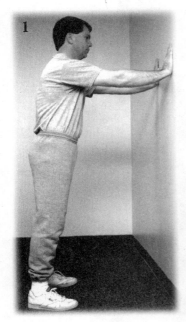

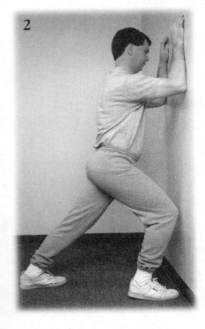

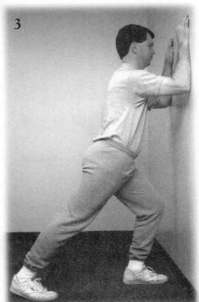

Calf stretch prepares muscles of the back and lower leg.

Modified hurdle stretch

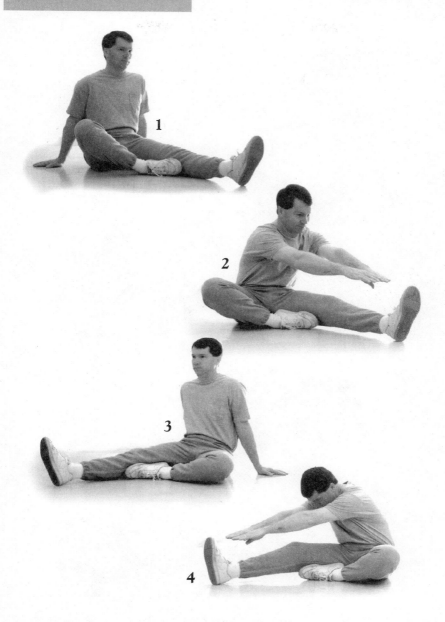

Modified hurdle stretch provides stretch and flexibility to upper back, groin, hamstrings, quadriceps, and calves.

Groin stretch

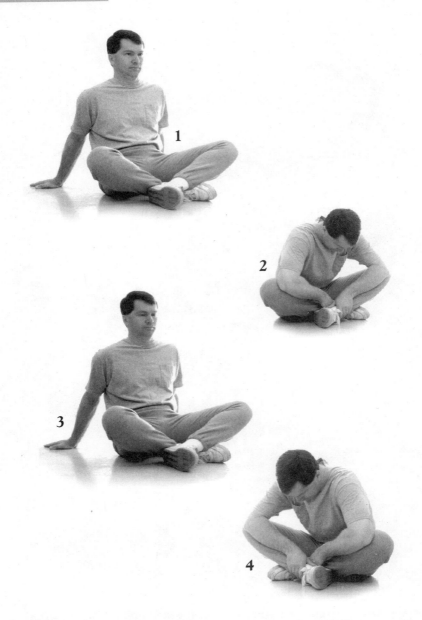

Groin stretch provides flexibility to the inner thigh and lower back.

Hamstring stretch

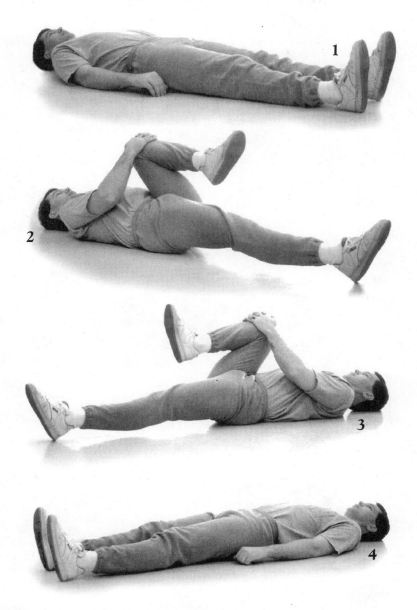

Hamstring stretch stretches lower back and hamstrings.

Modified sit up

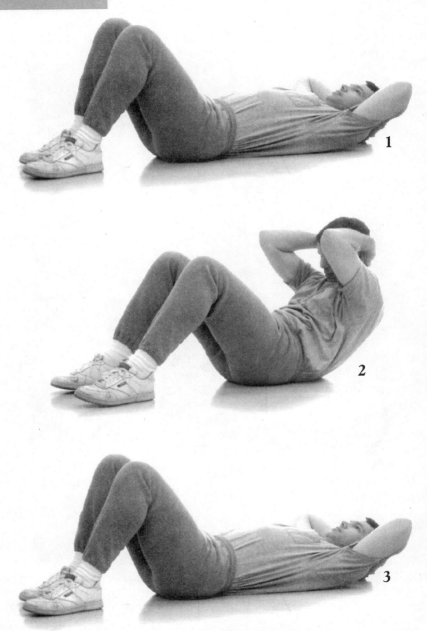

Modified sit-up strengthens muscles of the stomach wall.

CHAPTER 4

Food, Food, Food

As a young boy I would joyfully visit my dad's business. My mom would drive me the short distance and park behind his old building on a sandy Florida parking lot. Upon entering the store, most of the time I would stop to weigh myself on the heavy duty set of produce scales to see if I had gained any weight. I was small for my age and determined to put on some much needed poundage. After weighing, I would proceed through the swinging door and enter my dad's domain. It had clean pine shavings on the floor and a large walk-in cooler near the entry. A long row of refrigerated cases full of *good stuff* separated my dad's department from the rest of the store. My dad was an old-fashioned meat cutter. He would greet his customers wearing khaki pants, collared shirt, and a blood-stained apron. He would personally cut your choice of meat to perfection. Every child received something special from my dad every time they came to his store. He was a caring man and a wonderful provider for our family.

Being part-owner in a grocery store provided its own perks. We ate the best and were always assured by daddy that, "You'll never go hungry." Of course, eating well in those days meant plenty of red meat. The nutritionists of that period emphasized the need of a big chunk of red meat as the centerpiece of a well-rounded plate full of food. Whole milk was also the order of the day. I can remember that as a high schooler I would eat as many as five fattening meals and consume a full gallon of milk (168 grams of fat) in the course of each day. Later, as a college student and athlete majoring in physical education, I would never miss a meal. Breakfast, lunch, and supper would find me in the college cafeteria line loading up my tray. After devouring my meal, I would beg for any leftovers from those sitting at my table. Again, I assumed that this was a healthy diet. At the time, I was very strong and felt great. My physique, resulting from hundreds of hours of weight lifting, certainly gave no indication that I was injecting a potentially lethal combination of fat and cholesterol into my body. So I continued down the path of a confirmed coronary by-pass candidate.

I wish I knew then what I know now! My dietary habits would have been considerably different, and I may have bypassed by-pass surgery. This preacher is no *know-it-all* in regard to nutrition, but I have come to some definite, simple conclusions which, if heeded, could pay dividends in the future. Good eating habits now will play a significant role in preventing disease later. Most of us, however, wait until a health crisis such as a heart attack or cancer before we are willing to change our eating habits. Please don't be guilty of that serious mistake!

As I thought about how to get my point across on food, I came up with the following analogy. As preachers of the Word of God, we know that some things are not negotiable. For example, Adrian Rogers, dealing with the Ten Commandments, makes an important point. He says "The Ten Commandments are not accidental or incidental, they are fundamental. They are not obsolete, they are absolute." The world on the other hand has a different viewpoint. Ted Turner, the reprobate, media mogul, announced a few years ago that the Ten Commandments were obsolete and that they should be replaced with the *Ten Voluntary Initiatives. A U.S. News and World Report* article by John Leo spoke of the *Ten Tentative Suggestions.* That makes my blood boil! How about you? We should be dogmatic, emphatic, and enthusiastic about the eternal principles found in the inspired Word of God. No compromise is acceptable regarding *"Thus saith the Lord."*

But, on this issue of food's place in health and fitness, I get weary of those who think they have *the* answer. The *experts* on nutrition have problems agreeing on the perfect formula. The dieters argue with the vitamin/mineral supplement proponents; and they, in turn, cannot agree with the herbal-addicts. Sometimes, I want to throw my hands up in dismay when I hear so much information that contradicts. They remind me of the evolutionists!

So allow me to be somewhat less than dogmatic on this topic of food. Okay, I'll use a milquetoast phrase previously mentioned. Here are my Top Ten Tentative Suggestions on eating habits. These suggestions are not all that radical and can be incorporated into our basic family lifestyles.

Suggestion #1   Eat A Balanced Diet

My foremost recommendation concerning proper diet is to eat a wide variety of foods which includes a balance of many nutrients. Our bodies are created by the Lord to be finely tuned machines which must fuel up on the right combination of foods. Without doubt, a daily varied and balanced diet will do far more for your overall health than concentrating on certain foods or dietary supplements. God made such a wonderful variety of foods and He intends for us to enjoy eating. Unless you have a specific health problem, there is no need to totally give up your favorite foods. Temperance or self-control is the key. A diet that is effective and appropriate for everyone does not exist, but an excellent model for our daily diet is seen on the labels of many food products.

The United States Departments of Agriculture and Health and Human Services have provided a food pyramid. It provides a very attainable model for a healthy combination of foods. It includes the following: 6-11 servings of bread, cereal, rice, or pasta; 3-5 servings of vegetables; 2-4 servings of fruit, 2-3 servings of milk, yogurt, or cheese; 2-3 servings of meats, poultry, fish, dry beans, eggs, or nuts. And, of course, fats, sweets, and oils are to be used sparingly. Notice that this pyramid emphasizes complex carbohydrates. These are high in fiber and loaded with vitamins and minerals. The bread and cereal groups at the base of the pyramid should be a high priority in your diet. Fruits and veggies should come close behind as they contain no cholesterol and are almost always low in saturated fat. The dairy category should be the low fat or no fat variety. The meat group should be lean, small portions, and trimmed of excess fat. Chicken is much healthier with the skin removed, preferably before cooking, and cooked by methods other than deep frying. Fish is a tremendous choice whether fresh or frozen. Some cultures which eat lots of fish have lower rates of heart disease. Dry beans have high protein and are a good substitute for meat.

You, like me, may have a sweet tooth. You do not have to give up your sweets to be healthy. I do not intend to! Just be conscious of what you are eating. Think about the ingredients and the amount of calories, fat, and cholesterol you are consuming.

There is also a lot of hoopla today about vitamin and mineral supplements, making it a multi-million dollar industry. My family and I do take vitamins and minerals, but I am very concerned about the claims of toxicity from overdoses from the mega-vitamins. While it is probably true that our food supplies are not as nutritious because of additives, preservatives, and the depletion of soil quality, we must be careful not to swing to the other extreme. Again, I advise you to eat a well-balanced diet and consider reasonable amounts of absorbable supplements according to your individual needs. Experimentation with food varieties, vitamins, and minerals may be the key. If it works stick with it; if not, keep trying. You may also want to consult a knowledgeable physician or dietitian.

Suggestion #2   Achieve and Maintain a Desirable Body Weight

As I mentioned in the discussion of risk factors, "Approximately 30 percent of the American population has the distinction of being 20 percent above the designated, desirable body weight." That is the definition of obesity. Why are so many of us overweight, fat, and obese? It is because we consume far too many calories and fat grams. It takes little common sense to understand that we must burn more calories than we consume in order to lose weight. So the simple solution is to eat less, eat right, and exercise more. Stay away from bizarre diets which produce a yo-yo effect of weight loss and are potentially dangerous. Commit to a plan that achieves and maintains a desirable body weight.

The following formula was shared with me at the Portland Adventist Cardiac Rehab Center. This formula will give you an idea of what, and how much you can eat in order to lose and keep off excess weight. Take your ideal weight and multiply it by fifteen. That will give you your allotted calorie intake for the day. Then take that number and multiply it by .20. That will give you the allowable intake of calories from fat per day. Take that number and divide it by nine. That will give you your total number of fat grams per day. Sound complicated? It's not really. Here is the formula using an ideal body weight of 180.

Ideal body weight 180 x 15 = 2700 calories per day
Calories per day 2700 x .20 = 540 calories from fat per day
Calories from fat 540 divided by 9 = 60 total fat grams per day

This is the formula which can be used to determine the calories and fat allowance for a man. Your wife can use the same formula by simply changing the number fifteen to thirteen. Everything else remains the same.

It also stands to reason that if you are going to reduce your weight, you must consume less than what it would take to maintain your ideal body weight. Just remember, though, to go slow and steady in your weight loss program. A goal of a pound or two per week should be the maximum, as rapid weight loss could be hazardous to your health. Another suggestion is to subtract no more than 500 calories from your individual weight requirement. Again, if your weight loss is not gradual, if it is too abrupt, you could build up cravings and also resent your new lifestyle.

As you eat throughout the day, budget your calories and plan ahead. Work a food diary like a check book. The key is to come out at the end of the day without being overdrawn. I spent nine months with a food diary recording every calorie and fat gram I ate through-out the day. Now I know without a written record how I am doing. Some days I bounced a few calories/fat checks, but I kept my focus on the average. I can even give you my nine-month average — it was 2,435 daily average for calories and 19.36 average daily fat grams. I am slightly over these numbers now, but I keep it close to that ideal, and as a result my weight stays within a one- to three-pound variance.

It is important to be patient. Sometimes weight loss plateaus for a while. Just stay with it. Stay healthy and remain consistent. Don't weigh every day; once a week is fine. You can be your own personal trainer and keep your weight off without spending a fortune on weight loss programs.

Suggestion #3   Reduce Fat and Cholesterol

An excessive amount of fat in the diet not only contributes to heart disease, but to numerous forms of cancer and other deadly or debilitating maladies. Too much cholesterol increases the risk of atherosclerosis (the closing off of blood vessels, especially those sup-plying the heart muscle itself). Some fat is necessary for optimal health. It provides insulation, protection, stores energy, and trans-ports certain fat soluble vitamins. Likewise, cholesterol is essential to every cell in the body. But it is obvious that Americans take in too much dietary fat and cholesterol.

As I stated in the section on a balanced diet, unless there is a health problem, you do not have to totally give up your favorite foods, just reduce the portions and frequencies of them.

Nutrition studies generally recommended that fat intake total no more than 20 to 30 percent of total calorie consumption and that saturated fat be less than 10 percent. Cholesterol levels should be around 150-180 mg. per day for those having one or more risk factors and less than 200-300 mg. if no risk factors are involved. One study indicated that lowering the total cholesterol count by 25 percent could reduce the risk of heart attack by one-half. Yet, probably less than 10 percent of the population knows their cholesterol level.

Suggestion #4   Eat Often Each Day

This recommendation should be music to the diet junky's ears. Don't starve your body, feed it! Eating large meals, widely spread out through the day promotes weight gain and can increase cholesterol levels. On the other hand, frequent eating and vigorous exercise combine to step up metabolism and burn calories. Eat before you are starving. Nurse Olivia Rossi of Portland Cardiac Rehab says, "When it comes to hunger, like pain, keep ahead of it."

It is important not to skip meals unless, of course, you are fasting. It is also a very good idea to stop eating before you are full. This could have many healthy benefits. I start each day with a big, healthy breakfast that includes plenty of grains and fruit. I then, normally, eat a mid-morning snack around ten o'clock. Lunch is followed by a mid-afternoon snack, supper, and a night snack. This plan coupled with exercise has actually helped me tremendously in weight loss.

Now, I know this is going to upset some of your schedules, but you need to take the time to eat breakfast. After a night's rest you are ready physiologically to "break your fast." Your blood sugar is low and energy is needed for your busy day. As your mother told you, "Breakfast is the most important meal of the day." So eat that healthy breakfast and do like me — eat all day! Yum-yum!

Suggestion #5   Substitute Ingredients and Food Selections

A healthy diet is not a starvation exercise. You can eat a greater volume of food, thus satisfying your hunger by creative substitutions. There are many healthy cookbooks on the market which contain hundreds of tasty recipes so I'll not spend a lot of time on this section. Here are just a few major ideas.

First, in the area of ingredients replace lard, butter, bacon fat, etc. with fat substitutes. We have found Smart Beat, a product of Heart Beat Foods, and Lighter Bake made by Sunsweet to be good substitutes. Or you may want to just switch to a soft margarine in a tub. When cooking with oils, it's good to choose light vegetable oils that are highest in unsaturated fats. Examples are canola, safflower, sunflower, corn, and olive especially those in the spray containers.

It's important to use as little oil as possible because in spite of deceptive claims, all oils have fat. Use salad dressings that are low- or non-fat. A salad with fattening dressing is not part of a low fat/cholesterol diet. In all cooking, make it a practice to use low or non-fat ingredients and consider baking, broiling, grilling, boiling, or poaching instead of frying.

Consider these changes concerning overall food selections. Eat meatless meals a few times each week. Examples could be pastas, beans, or rice. Our kids seldom ask, "Where's the beef?" in these types of meals. In fact, some of these dishes are their favorites. Remember, protein is protein, with or without the fat.

Milk is another big category. Earlier I shared that my diet when I was growing up would contain up to 168 grams of fat per day just from milk. Today it is zero. We switched from whole milk (8 grams per serving) to 2 percent (5 grams) to 1 percent (3 grams) to — "Wait a minute, I'm not drinking blue milk!" Skim milk has come a long way from that colored water-looking stuff. Now skim milk can be produced with additives which take care of the thickness problem. It may be marketed under several labels. Here in Oregon it is called ultra-skim or skim deluxe. It passes my palatability test and I really endorse it.

Cheese is another story. Most diet cheese tastes like diet cheese! Yuk! I can't help you much here. (My wife's note: "Non-fat cheese used in casseroles tastes fine. He eats it all the time without complaining. What he doesn't know, doesn't hurt him.") Let me know if you discover a tasty alternative.

Eggs — no problem. I sure can't stand the egg substitutes, but get rid of some of the yolk and you get rid of a lot of cholesterol. We, on occasion, will put in several egg whites and throw in a yolk for color and taste. Some people use straight egg whites. The result — no fat and no cholesterol.

Snacks and desserts are also important in my book. Again, the key is a healthy addition to your food intake. Instead of ice cream, go for low- or non-fat frozen yogurt, ice milk, or sherbert. But be sure to check the label to see what you are getting. There are many low-fat snacks such as pretzels, crackers, fruit bars, yogurt, and even fruit. I suppose my greatest weakness in food is chocolate. Milk chocolate is almost completely off my diet, but Nestle's *Quik* is my choice. It only has one-half gram of fat per serving and is 99 percent caffeine free. Can you believe I usually have a chocolate milkshake before bedtime? With skim milk, non-fat frozen yogurt, and Nestle's *Quik*, the total fat count is still one-half gram. So, Preacher, substitution and food selections can make a measurable impact on your nutritional needs.

Suggestion #6   Learn to Read and Understand Labels

Some books on the subject of labels are very detailed, but let me give you just a few pointers. Since 1992, there have been some real upgrades regarding nutritional labels on most food products. You must understand what these facts mean.

Remember to judge your nutritional totals from the first piece of information listed on the label. Are you eating the same amount as the serving size? That will make a big difference! If you are eating twice the recommended serving size, you must double the rest of the categories. Look at the total calories as well as the calories from fat. Know the total grams of fat as well as what kind of fat it contains. Saturated fat is the one which sends up red flags. Be concerned about the cholesterol, sodium, carbohydrates, sugars, and the amount of dietary fiber. It does not take long to glance at the food labels and it will certainly be well worth your time.

Suggestion #7   Drink Water

We have been very fortunate to have had a very good water source in each of our homes, but I have never been a big water consumer. Like many other things, I drink water because it is good for me. I haven't quite achieved the FDA recommended six to eight glasses per day, but I have certainly improved. If you do not have an adequate water source, try bottled water. If you still have difficulty, try a bit of lemon or lime in your water.

Water is certainly important during your exercise periods. It is the best diuretic to clean out impurities and hydrate your body which is made up of 70 percent water.

Since my heart surgery I have felt a little weak at times, especially between Sunday School and the worship service. Recently, I have tried to correct that by drinking about sixteen ounces of a sports drink. It seems to give me that little extra boost of energy to make it through the day. While that's not quite the same as drinking water, I thought it might help some of you.

Suggestion #8   Limit Caffeine, Salt, Sugar, and Preservatives

Caffeine is a chemical substance which should be limited especially by those who have a family history of heart disease, high blood pressure, or who suffer adverse affects from its use. How much caffeine you can safely use varies according to your sensitivity. But in general, the more you take in, the more agitated you will become. That fact along with other possible side effects should send red flags up about caffeine.

Excessive salt consumption may elevate blood pressure in some people. High sodium content, especially in processed foods, should be a real concern. Check labels and lean toward those foods which contain low sodium or salt. Most of us do not even need the salt shaker on the table since most foods are well seasoned in preparation. You may want to experiment with other seasonings such as herbs, spices, onions, garlic, pepper, or even lemon juice. Choose salt substitutes or lite salt. We have found Morton Lite Salt with half the sodium of table salt to be the best alternative.

With preservatives, the less the better. So much goes into food today that it's hard to avoid them. One writer stated, "Put nothing in your mouth that you can't pronounce." I'm not that fanatical, but it is food for thought.

Let me now say a word about sugar. What can I say? I love it! But that, too, in excess can be dangerous. Sugar, though it has only seventeen calories per level teaspoon, can pack a lot of calories in a small quantity. Soft drinks, candy, and many desserts can run up your calorie content in a big hurry. Sugar also promotes tooth decay.

Suggestion #9   Avoid Fad Diets and Quick Fixes

Diets are a way of life for millions. Diets may help you shed pounds quickly, but usually those pounds are gained back with a few extra to spare. Quick-fix programs can cause chemical imbalances and result in dangerous medical conditions. Please stay away from crash diets and diet pills. Starvation diets cause fat cells to shrink and the dieter will appear thinner, but when "normal" eating resumes, the cells will grow larger. (Fat cells can expand by nine times their original size.) Instead, it is wise to balance your diet and eat sensibly for life. This can become a reality through changes in attitude and behavior. Enjoy food, but don't make each meal an exercise in indulgence or denial.

Fasting is a great spiritual exercise with the added benefit of cleansing the body and developing godly discipline. Jesus commanded fasting for spiritual reasons, but never gave it as a method of weight loss.

So please, Preacher, don't be conned into these ridiculous diet schemes. Enjoy food, eat right, and exercise self-control.

Suggestion #10   Use Wisdom When Eating Out

Try to go to restaurants that offer a wide variety of foods and that will prepare it the way you request. Be bold enough to ask for specifics when you order. Some eating establishments have American Heart Association Heart Health menu choices. Even fast food places can be a source of healthy food if you know what you are looking for. My daughter, Krista, worked at a local McDonald's restaurant. She received discounted food as a benefit of her employment, but even at age seventeen she is health conscious. We have nutritional charts from McDonald's, Taco Bell, and TCBY. We also have a book that gives calorie counts and fat grams for items from dozens of restaurants. You do not have to be a rocket scientist to eat heart smart!

Here are some pointers that will help you when dining out.

• At fast food restaurants, choose grilled chicken without mayonnaise; grab a few french fries, not an entire order. Share the rest, because they are loaded with fat. Eat frozen yogurt or a healthy muffin for dessert.

• Go with big salads with low-fat or non-fat dressings on the side. You can dip your fork in the dressing, then in the salad for the minimum amount of dressing.

• Request baked, broiled, or grilled meat rather than fried.

• Choose baked potato (without butter) instead of french fries. Consider rice or pasta. Those are good choices.

• Avoid creamed foods, sour cream, foods cooked in gravy, cheese spreads, mayo-based salads, and real bacon bits.

• Give steamed vegetables a try. Of course, leave off butter or cheese.

• Try to live without the fattening desserts. If you do order one, split it with your wife.

Church-wide fellowships also give the preacher another area of concern. Those can really be detrimental to your waistline and, of course, are a real temptation to *fudge*. At the next fellowship, exercise your biblical self-control and refrain from pigging out. If you do not want to hurt feelings, just get a taste of all those wonderful dishes. Why not bring your own contribution? Our church has a lot of healthy choices at fellowship time, so it's no real problem for me. On occasion, I will indulge in a small portion of a fattening dish. Our folk know my situation and yours should know your commitment to eating right. You'll find that they usually understand.

When invited out to eat or to a member's home, use your own good common sense. You do not have to compromise your health to please everyone. Be polite, sensible, and self-controlled. You'll be just fine.

So, Preacher, how will you respond to these Ten Tentative Suggestions? They will make a real difference in your health.

CHAPTER 5

Stressed Out

Preachers are, no doubt, some of the most stressed out people on the planet. Should that be true? No! But is it true? You better believe it! I'm not a doctor, nor the son of a doctor, but I can almost guarantee that stress played a significant role in my coronary heart disease leading to a heart attack. Lack of stress management could be the single most overlooked contributing risk factor influencing heart disease.

To be honest with you, I am still somewhat a victim of unmanaged stress. Completing this book even added to my stress level. I have researched this subject, have implemented many of the principles that I am sharing with you, but for some reason, I am still usually high strung and have to shut down at times just to keep from going over the edge. This has been especially the case since having bypass surgery. Jennifer says it's just my "thorn in the flesh." I would love to hear from some of you preachers who identify with my situation.

To cover this subject of stress management, I need to explore four important points.

Defining Stress

Stress is certainly an unavoidable part of our everyday life. Stress is caused by any external influence that interferes with our normal mind and body rhythms. It manifests itself in a multitude of *fight, fright,* or *flight* responses. One doctor states that *stress* is "the non-specific response of the body to any demand." Stress can be the result of a positive or negative situation. It may be good and pleasant or bad and unpleasant. The body does not differentiate, it simply responds to a change in normal activity or even thought patterns. Stress is a part of this fearfully and wonderfully made human body and so we must learn to live with it or rather manage it.

Detecting Stress

Our bodies respond to stress by pumping extra adrenaline into the bloodstream to assist us in dealing with emergencies in a quick and efficient manner. Stress can be detected easiest in Type A personalities, of which most preachers can be classified. Type A's are gripped with a sense of urgency, trying to cram too much into too little time. Type A's have trouble relaxing and many times are workaholics. This personality can be plagued by obsessive-compulsive tendencies and in some studies have shown twice the risk of coronary heart disease.

Unmanaged stress or distress can affect the body in several ways. The heart may race or palpitate, breathing problems such as hyperventilation may be present, dizziness and lightheadedness may also result. The digestive system may respond by indigestion, nausea, constipation, or diarrhea. Our bodies and minds may respond with symptoms of depression or even panic attacks.

To really identify unmanaged stress as well as characteristics of the Type A personality, I have broken the symptoms down into two categories. The first category consists of the physical manifestations and the second category contains behavioral characteristics. No one suffers from all of these symptoms, but it will at least help you get a handle on your situation.

Physical Manifestations
- Headaches
- Tense muscles in neck, shoulders, back, jaw, etc.
- Tingling in arms and hands
- Nervous tics
- Trembling
- Cold hands and feet
- Excessive sweating

Behavioral Characteristics
- Impatience
- Constant rushing

- Inability to sit long
- Speaking and eating fast
- Irritability
- Nervous, anxious, or constant worry
- Highly competitive, hating to lose
- Overbearing
- Excitable, high strung
- Expecting too much (from self and others)
- Insomnia
- Fidgeting
- Excessive fatigue

These are some factors to look for in detecting stress. It is very important to identify our stressors as well as recognize the dangers of the unmanaged stress. That leads us to the next major category.

The Dangers of Unmanaged Stress

Let's first establish the fact that not all stress is bad. Stress can greatly benefit us by getting us moving and keeping us alert to real dangers in life. Stress can aid us in completing difficult tasks and even contribute to high achievement. But there is a danger from stress overload. Normally, stress operates in an ebb and flow. We have periods of high adrenalin arousal, then we back off and rest. Our bodies and minds can potentially withstand great amounts of stress, but if it is overly prolonged or too intense, illness (both physically and mentally) may be inevitable. Some people may feel little or no discomfort until damaging results appear. So be alert, but remember, it's not the outside circumstances or people (the stressors) that are the dangers, rather it's how we react on a continuous basis.

Dealing With Stress

We cannot totally eliminate stress from our lives, but we can control our reactions to the stressors and thus lessen its adverse effects. We can view change (a big part of stress) as a challenge and transform stress into a positive experience. Consider the following suggestions.

Look to the Lord and His Word. Consider Jesus, the author and finisher of our faith.This is certainly the place to start. If anyone had a right to be stressed to the limit, it was our Lord. He was fully God, but He was also fully man. Remember the balanced life he lived and the practical side of His ministry. He had his disciples as

His supportive circle (though sometimes they were anything but supportive). And on occasion, He withdrew in solitude for spiritual refreshment. *"And he said unto them, Come ye yourselves apart into a desert place, and rest a while: for there were many coming and going, and they had no leisure so much as to eat"* (Mark 6:31).

The Word of God deals very forcefully with stressors such as anger, worry, fear, and guilt. The Lord gives us some wonderful scriptures about how to deal with these and other areas of our personal lives. Philippians 4 is one of the greatest passages in all the Word of God in dealing with worry and anxiety. In verse 4, it tells us to *"rejoice in the Lord alway: and again I say, Rejoice."* It emphasizes moderation or self-control in verse 5 and then deals directly with the sin of worry in verse 6. Paul said, *"Be careful* (anxious care or worry) *for nothing; but in every thing by prayer and supplication with thanksgiving let your requests be made known unto God."* Good counsel — rejoice, be under control by the Spirit, don't worry about anything, but pray about everything. The result is found in verse 7, *"And the peace of God, which passeth all understanding, shall keep your hearts and minds through Christ Jesus."* God pulls no punches in these verses. He goes to the heart of the problem, which is a problem of the heart. Verse 8 then tells us to keep our thoughts on that which is true, honest, pure, lovely, things that are of a good report, virtuous, and praiseworthy. Without a doubt, these are some of the most fantastic verses in all the Bible to help deal with unmanaged stress.

Other scriptures deal with our relationships. Face it; we can have some of the same problems as the folk in the pews. So we must deal head-on with bitterness, forgiveness, acceptance, and a whole host of interpersonal relationships. Focus on the Lord. We really have no business failing to practice what we preach. So preacher brethren, let's look to the Lord and His Word.

Practice the three A's. The three A's are alter, adapt, and anticipate. You may have the ability to alter your situation or surroundings to reduce stress. You may have to be more assertive and learn to say no. Remember, it is not God's will for you to do everything! So alter. It may be necessary for you to adapt your attitude or your activities. Then, you need to anticipate. Plan how to handle people and situations in a loving, scriptural way. Cultivate the ability to deal with problem people and how to choose your words wisely. Also remember Proverbs 9:8 tells us that no amount of words will help some people. It states, *"Reprove not a scorner, lest he hate thee."* Sometimes our counsel is simply casting our pearls before swine. So, alter, adapt, and anticipate.

Have the proper perspective. We often make mountains out of mole hills and worry about things that never happen. Remember, *worry* is "assuming responsibilities that God never intended you to have." It is paying interest on tomorrow's problems which may never happen. So, have the proper perspective on life's problems. (Oops! I meant challenges!)

While flying into Dallas International Airport recently, I observed the thousands of homes below, and it gave me a better perspective on my own situation. God sees the big picture, so keep your eyes on Him, not on your surroundings. That will give you the proper perspective.

Set realistic goals. God has a potential for every preacher. It is His work and His ministry. Goal setting is important, but be sure you are getting your vision from God and His Word. Young ministers may aspire to be the next D.L. Moody or Charles H. Spurgeon. God wants us to set our sights high, but you are who you are, and are not called to become carbon copies of another pastor, preacher, missionary, or evangelist. If we do not set realistic, God-given goals, we are setting ourselves up for a big fall and a colossal mid-life crisis. We may even become disillusioned and eventually become a castaway in God's work.

Acknowledge your problem and identify your stressors. You may have to come to grips with the fact that you are a Type A personality. If not, you might at least possess some Type A characteristics which could be harmful. Write down your stressors and consider counseling with a competent fellow preacher. A Stanford University report that was done several years ago revealed that heart attack victims who received *Type A counseling* had more than 50 percent fewer recurring heart attacks than those who received no counseling. Of course, there are also some very good books on this subject.

Be wise in your counseling. Preachers are certainly in demand to counsel others. It is an awesome privilege and a serious ministry task. But as we counsel, we must stick to the Word of God, give the appropriate counsel coupled with prayer, and then leave the results to God. Do not feel you must change the person. Just as in our soul winning experiences, it is God that gives the increase and God that changes the heart. Be careful not to become too overwhelmed with other people's problems and do not take your work home at night.

The preceding thoughts thus far have dealt with mental, spiritual, and emotional exercises. Now, we will deal with some physical helps.

Eat right and exercise. Chapters three and four of this book deal with these two important areas. Remember, our fitness and health in the areas of nutrition and exercise have a direct relationship to our stress management.

Slow down and relax. Type A's think rapidly about many subjects at once. We keep a lot of ideas churning away, and sometimes, even in our sleep we are still revved up. We must learn to slow down and change our thinking habits. We must also change our attitudes and behavior.

Relaxation techniques for counteracting stress-related symptoms are important to develop. Set a priority to relax hourly, daily, and weekly. Let's observe these in reverse order. First, we need to relax weekly. God made us to take a day of rest. No, Sunday certainly does not qualify. How many preachers would say Sunday is their day of rest? Just the opposite is true. We need a day away from the problems and challenges of the ministry. (Not a day away from God, just your realm of ministry.) The church I pastor is very considerate concerning my day off. I take Monday off, and unless someone dies or the equivalent, I try to stay unavailable. Occasionally, this rest day may be interrupted, but that is the rare exception and not the rule.

Second, we need to rest daily. Take at least thirty minutes each day to nap or just relax with no outside disturbance. Toward the end of my workday afternoons I spend at least thirty minutes either in a dark classroom or at home away from everyone. I breathe deeply and stretch from the end of my fingertips to the tips of my toes. I then close my eyes, systematically relax my entire body, and tune out the world. I think pleasant thoughts of calm restful places I have been. Sometimes, I go over portions of God's Word. I stay relaxed until I am rested and calmed down. I get up slowly and gradually resume my activities. Daily relaxation allows the body to recharge and balance the bad effects of stress. We should relax even on non-stressful days.

Third, we should relax hourly. I will have to be honest with you on this point. It is so easy for me to get caught up in my work that I do not move until I have completed it. I have, however, made it a practice to take breaks and walk around for a few minutes to wind down from what I am immersed in. This can and should be done regularly, and if possible, hourly. It all adds up weekly, daily, and hourly.

We also need to take planned, relaxing, not rushed, vacations. Remember, even Jesus took the time to come apart for a time.

Listen to your body. When symptoms of distress are present in our lives, we need to listen and take appropriate action. When I experience arm tingling, hyperventilation, a drawing up in the lower rib area, or an overall feeling of panic, I know it's time to shut down and relax. Earlier in this chapter I listed some symptoms of prolonged or intense stress. When you recognize these symptoms, they should be addressed as soon as possible. Listen to that body of yours because God placed an early warning system in you which surpasses any modern technology.

Get plenty of rest and sleep. I touched briefly on this when I spoke concerning relaxation, but it is so important. The human body requires rest and adequate sleep to be restored and refreshed. Doctor Archibald Hart in his book, *Adrenalin and Stress,* has devoted an entire chapter to sleep and another chapter to relaxation. I highly recommend this book. Dr. Hart is Dean of the Graduate School of Psychology and Professor of Psychology at Fuller Theological Seminary in Pasadena, California. He theorizes that we need much more sleep than commonly thought, and that much research to the contrary in the past was significantly flawed. Sleeping does not shorten your life! So Preacher, get a good night's sleep consistently — not what someone else needs, but what you need. Take many mini-vacations of rest each day. Also, avoid taking sleeping aids or tranquilizers. Very rarely will these additives be needed if we follow some sensible techniques. Dr. Hart's book is filled with usable advice.

Organize your time. Identify time wasters and break big projects into jobs of manageable size. Prioritize your workload into essential, important, and trivial. Do dreaded tasks early in the day. Allow some extra time before and after appointments or tasks just to catch your breath and to calm down. Learn to say no, and learn to do one thing at a time. And above all, learn to delegate responsibilities. You will accomplish much more and will be following some good, biblical advice.

Enjoy a non-stress hobby. Get involved in something you enjoy doing, and, thus, get your mind off your work for a time. This could be a family activity or an individual hobby.

Avoid unnecessary conflict. Notice that I said *unnecessary* conflict. By its very nature, our ministries sometime involve conflict and unpleasant confrontations. And we must be busy, earnestly contending for the faith. But a requirement for a pastor is found in I Timothy 3:3. It says a bishop should be *"no striker."* That means not to be in the business of looking for a fight. We have enough God-given battle zones to occupy us without looking for more.

I have a real problem dealing with injustice in the world. Sometimes, I act as God's policeman trying to right every wrong. I have nearly gotten into serious trouble sticking my prophetic nose into situations with a fleshly attitude. Philippians 2:15 has helped me deal with that problem. Look that up and pray that we might all constantly apply it.

Get up earlier. I am not contradicting my advice about getting enough sleep. However, I am saying preachers probably need to go to bed earlier than the average person. We need to go to bed and schedule enough sleep time in order to get up early to spend time with God. Also, this will avoid most interruptions.

Maintain a sense of humor. We need to learn to laugh at ourselves. Laughter is wonderful medicine. Remember the wise man's words in Proverbs 17:22, *"A merry heart doeth good like a medicine: but a broken spirit drieth the bones."* Good, godly humor and a happy attitude will do much for our physical, emotional, and spiritual well-being. We need to be serious about our calling and work, but also radiate the joy of the Lord. According to Nehemiah 8:10, *"The joy of the LORD is your strength."*

Don't put up with things that do not work. Inanimate objects can drive some folks up the wall. I have wanted to murder lawn mowers and other mechanical objects that don't work. Fix it or throw it away!

Don't use negative self-talk. Avoid negative words in your self-talk, like *can't, always,* and *never.* Many times we are our own worst critics and enemies. Be careful about discouraging words and heed Philippians 4:8.

Don't rely on memory alone. It is so easy to forget important appointments, responsibilities, or even prayer requests. When someone asks me to do or remember something, I usually respond, "I'll write that down!" Then I follow through. My memory is certainly not reliable. Write down your list of priorities.

Restrict caffeine. This can be especially important in sensitive people. Each of us is different. Remember, listen to your body!

Be concerned about your outward appearance. How you look has an impact on how you feel. Remember your calling.

Hopefully, these suggestions will help. We are all different. What works for someone else, may not work for you. Experiment! If something does not work, try something else. Damaging effects of stressors can be minimized.

May God bless you, preacher brother. My prayer for you is the same which John related in His third epistle, *"Beloved, I wish above all things that thou mayest prosper and be in health, even as thy soul prospereth"* (III John 2).

6

From the Heart of the Helper

Author's Note: I have asked my wife Jennifer to make a contribution to this book. Here she shares from her perspective and experience. It will be especially helpful to the preacher's wife.

"He'll be okay, Jennifer; he's just missing you." This was the general thought of my family when James called saying that he had been diagnosed with pleurisy, but wasn't getting any better.

The Lord had enabled me to be present at the birth of my second granddaughter, Hannah Elizabeth Lea. This was a very special time for me since I was unable to be with my daughter Kari when her first daughter, Sarah Kaitlyn, was born. (All you grandmothers will understand what I mean!)

Why did James have to get sick and make me start feeling guilty about leaving him with our other three children? He really knows how to spoil a party! Little did I know what was really happening back home in Oregon, or what was about to happen to change our lives.

After returning home, my concern began to grow as James did not get better. *Yoo-hoo! James, I'm home now; it's time to get well!* After all, wasn't he just missing me? His chest pains were getting worse and more frequent. James could not walk to the end of our block without pain, and it even exhausted him to take a shower.

Any physical exertion brought pain.

He was due to leave for a church growth conference in Texas, and I had big question marks in my mind about whether he should go. I suggested (I have to use the word *suggested* in order to sound submissive, but it was more like a command!) that he see a cardiologist before he left on that trip. After the examination, the cardiologist's *command* was to cancel the Texas trip and to not do anything stressful. James was a time bomb waiting to explode.

Against the doctor's advice, my husband preached the next day to a very attentive audience — 195 people! It was Friend Day and our congregation had doubled that Sunday.

The next few days were tense. It was hard for me to let James out of my sight. I knew in my heart that God wasn't going to take my husband from me, but there was a little part of me that was thinking, *What if He does? What would I do? Where would I go?* I didn't know the answers to these questions (and I still don't), so I refused to think about them. I knew that I needed to be an encouragement to James and to be strong for him. This was no time for a pity party.

The day of the surgery (April 1) we awoke to what we at first thought was an April Fool's joke — my birdbath was gone! (This wasn't just *any* birdbath. The ladies of our church had given me this for my fortieth birthday, and it was my pride and joy! It took at least two people to lift it.) If it had been stolen on any other day, I would have cried for a week. But this day was different.

A birdbath was the least of my worries. At the end of the day, I was truly thankful that it was my birdbath that had been taken away from me and not my husband. The birdbath was replaced, but no one could take James' place!

Eight hours passed from the time James was rolled in to be prepped for surgery until the doctor came out to tell me that all was well. Needless to say, that was one of the longest days of my life. Four dear church members sat with me in the waiting room most of that day. Of course, I know there was an unseen Friend waiting with me also.

It is very important for a spouse to understand the trauma that has just taken place in her husband's life and to also realize that medication alters personality. I found out very quickly that I needed to think before I spoke. I first blundered by telling him the day after surgery that the doctor had discovered evidence of a previous heart attack. The look on his face told me everything. I quickly added, "But it was a mild one and there wasn't much damage at all!" Since James and I have always shared openly with one another about everything, I did not think about the impact those words would have on him. James had gone into surgery thinking that he had caught his condition early so that he would not have any heart damage. *Heart attack* were not words that he wanted to hear.

The next sticky situation came when James wanted me to read the Bible to him and he accused me of skipping some verses. I knew not to argue.

It became evident to me that for the next few weeks I would have to be very sensitive to the Lord's leading. James' emotions were up and down. He might be crying one minute and laughing uncontrollably the next. The only place he could sleep was the couch, so I brought my sleeping bag to the living room floor. I even spoon-fed him *Jell-O* in the middle of the night. (This all reminded me of having a newborn baby!)

Since he could not drive, I had to be free to take him wherever he wanted to go. He began going to the office for an hour at a time two weeks after surgery. He even did a funeral exactly two weeks after his surgery date. It was not an easy task to keep him down. I'll have to say that by the end of six weeks, the only thing that *really* bothered me was being his chauffeur. He was not a good backseat driver.

For several years, I had considered our family to be very health conscious. We stayed away from fried foods, and James and I walked three days a week. I am very fortunate that James *wants* to be healthy and is willing to make the sacrifices needed to be healthy. Some people with coronary heart disease are not willing to do that, endangering their lives and bringing grief to their families. (We all should be willing to take good care of the bodies God has given us.)

Two months after surgery James began to keep a record of every calorie and fat gram that he ate. My daughter, Krista, and I decided to make it a family project, so I bought each of us a little notebook and a calorie and fat counting book. It added fun to having to do without by seeing who had the least amount of calories and fat for the day. Krista usually won.

I really did not have to quit cooking our favorite dishes. I just learned to make substitutions. I learned to bake and grill instead of fry. I used egg whites and applesauce in muffins and cakes, instead of whole eggs and oil. We began drinking non-fat milk instead of 2 percent milk. I bought fat-free cheeses. We even learned to eat meatless meals and didn't have any withdrawal pains at all! Chicken is our main dish most of the time, but I will occasionally buy a very lean cut of beef or pork, and sometimes fish. Grains and pastas are wonderful additions to a meal. The whole secret is being willing to work together as a family. Our two younger children, Justin and Jenna, don't seem to mind too much either. They still get hot dogs (fat-free), hamburgers (extra lean and the meat scrambled in order to use less), and pizza (I even make a low-fat pizza!).

Our three-days-a-week walks turned into a six-days-a-week routine. I learned to include this in my daily schedule right along with sleeping, eating, and devotions. James wanted to lose twenty pounds as well as recondition his heart. Our walks started slowly for the first six weeks. James would walk with his hand over his heart. I told him that people were either going to think he was very patriotic, or that he was on the verge of a heart attack.

The wonderful thing about all of this is that I have lost weight and inches, too. (The family that exercises together, loses weight together!) Our walking also gives us thirty-five minutes each day of each other's undivided attention. We can share our joys or our burdens. An on-looker might think we are two kids out playing, when at a certain point we race to see who can touch the green dot on the blue sign first. Of course, James wins every time. (I have to let him win, you know.) Recently, I read that 94 percent of couples that begin an exercise program together, were still going a year later. We can testify to that! Encouragement and accountability are very important to a healthy exercise program.

The spouse's support is immensely essential to a preacher husband's well-being, whether he has coronary heart disease or not. Your husband relies on you emotionally and physically. God has placed you where you are to be a completer to your husband so that he can be the man of God that God has called him to be. Whether it is insisting that he go for his needed check-up, seeing that he eats healthy meals, joining him in an exercise program, or seeing to it that your home is a stress-free haven where your husband can unwind after a stress-filled day, *you can make a difference in the heart of your preacher!*